Behavior Change
Log Book
and
Wellness Journal

SECOND EDITION

PEARSON

Boston Columbus Indianapolis New York San Francisco Upper Saddle River
Amsterdam Cape Town Dubai London Madrid Milan Munich Paris Montréal Toronto
Delhi Mexico City São Paulo Sydney Hong Kong Seoul Singapore Taipei Tokyo

Executive Editor: Sandra Lindelof
Assistant Editor: Meghan Zolnay
Development Director: Barbara Yien
Managing Editor: Deborah Cogan
Associate Production Project Manager: Megan Power
Production Management, Composition, and Interior Design: Integra
Cover Design: Derek Bacchus
Manufacturing Buyer: Stacey Weinberger
Executive Marketing Manager: Neena Bali
Cover Photo Credits: Salad: NataliTerr/Fotolia; Tissue Box: Martin Green/Fotolia; Yoga Man: i love images/Fotolia; Bicycle helmet: vencav/fotolia; Cigarette: Nikolai Sorokin/Fotolia; Piggy Bank: robynmac/Fotolia; Recycling Bags: cerbi/Fotolia; Sunglasses/suntan lotion: caimacanul/Fotolia; Condom: Skogas/Fotolia; Espresso: Designer_Andrea/Fotolia; Alarm Clock: Ever/Fotolia; Pillows: karam miri/Fotolia; Sneakers & Water Bottle: onepony/Fotolia; Apple: xiangdong Li/Fotolia; Fitness Trainer: Ariwasabi/Fotolia; Dumbbells: blueee/Fotolia; Bicycle: Darko Zivkovic/Fotolia

1 2 3 4 5 6 7 8 9 10 11—BRR—15 14 13 12

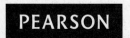

www.pearsonhighered.com

ISBN 10:   0-321-80317-5
ISBN 13: 978-0-321-80317-7

Table of Contents

1 Assess Yourself

This section of the Behavior Change Log Book will help you to prepare for behavior change by assessing your current health behaviors.

HOW HEALTHY ARE YOU?

Although we all recognize the importance of being healthy, it can be a challenge to sort out which behaviors are most likely to cause problems or which ones pose the greatest risk. Before you decide where to start, it is important to look at your current health status. Think carefully about where you believe you are today in each of the health dimensions. Rate your health status in each of the following dimensions by choosing the number that comes closest to describing the way you are most of the time.

Your Current Health Status

Point Scale: Very Poor = 1, Poor = 2, Average = 3, Good = 4, Excellent = 5

Physical Health	1	2	3	4	5
Social Health	1	2	3	4	5
Emotional Health	1	2	3	4	5
Environmental Health	1	2	3	4	5
Spiritual Health	1	2	3	4	5
Intellectual Health	1	2	3	4	5

After completing the above section, how would you rate your overall health?

_____

_____

Which area(s), if any, do you think you should work on improving?

_____

_____

If you were to ask your closest friends how healthy they think you are, which area(s) do you think they would say you need to improve?

_____

_____

Assessing Your Dimensions of Health

By completing the following assessment, you will have a clearer picture of health areas in which you excel and those that could use some work. Taking this assessment will also help you to reflect on components of health that you may not have thought about.

Answer each question, then total your score for each section and fill it in on the Personal Checklist at the end of the assessment for a better sense of your health profile. Think about the behaviors that influenced your score in each category. Would you like to change any of them?

Each of the categories in this questionnaire is an important aspect of the total dimensions of health, but this is not a substitute for the advice of a qualified health care provider. Consider scheduling a thorough physical examination by a licensed physician or setting up an appointment with a mental health counselor at your school if you need help making a behavior change.

For each of the following, indicate how often you think the statements describe you.

Physical Health

Point Scale: 1 = Never, 2 = Rarely, 3 = Some of the time, 4 = Usually or always

1. I am happy with my body size and weight. _____
2. I engage in vigorous exercises such as brisk walking, jogging, swimming, or running for at least 30 minutes per day, 3–4 times per week. _____
3. I do exercises designed to strengthen my muscles and increase endurance at least 2 times per week. _____
4. I do stretching, limbering, and balance exercises such as yoga, Pilates, or tai chi to increase my body awareness and control and increase my overall physical health. _____
5. I feel good about the condition of my body and would be able to respond to most demands placed upon it. _____
6. I get at least 7–8 hours of sleep each night. _____
7. I try to add moderate activity to each day, such as taking the stairs instead of the elevator and walking instead of driving whenever I can. _____
8. My immune system is strong, and my body heals itself quickly when I get sick or injured. _____
9. I have lots of energy and can usually get through the day without being overly tired. _____
10. I listen to my body; when there is something wrong, I try to make adjustments to heal it or seek professional advice. _____

Total score for this section: _____

Social Health

Point Scale: 1 = Never, 2 = Rarely, 3 = Some of the time, 4 = Usually or always

1. When I meet people, I feel good about the impression I make on them. _____
2. I am open and honest and get along well with others. _____
3. I participate in a wide variety of social activities and enjoy being with people who are different from me. _____
4. I try to be a "better person" and decrease behaviors that have caused problems in my interactions with others. _____
5. I get along well with members of my family. _____
6. I am a good listener. _____
7. I am open and accessible to a loving and responsible relationship. _____
8. I have someone I can talk to about my private feelings. _____

9. I consider the feelings of others and do not act in hurtful or selfish ways. _____

10. I try to see the good in my friends and do whatever I can to support them and help them feel good about themselves. _____

Total score for this section: _____

Emotional Health

Point Scale: 1 = Never, 2 = Rarely, 3 = Some of the time, 4 = Usually or always

1. I find it easy to laugh, cry, show emotions like love, fear, and anger, and try to express these in positive, constructive ways. _____

2. I avoid using alcohol or other drugs as a means of helping me forget or cope with my problems. _____

3. When facing a particularly challenging situation, I tend to view the glass as "half full" rather than "half empty" and perceive problems as opportunities for growth. _____

4. When I am angry, I try to let others know in non-confrontational and non-hurtful ways and try to resolve issues rather than stewing about them. _____

5. I try not to worry unnecessarily and to talk about my feelings, fears, and concerns rather than letting them become chronic issues. _____

6. I recognize when I am stressed and take steps to relax through exercise, quiet time, or other calming activities. _____

7. I feel good about myself and believe others like me for who I am. _____

8. I try not to be too critical or judgmental of others and try to understand differences or quirks that I note in others. _____

9. I am flexible and adapt or adjust to change in a positive way. _____

10. My friends regard me as a stable, emotionally well-adjusted person whom they can trust and rely on for support. _____

Total score for this section: _____

Environmental Health

Point Scale: 1 = Never, 2 = Rarely, 3 = Some of the time, 4 = Usually or always

1. I am concerned about environmental pollution and actively try to preserve and protect natural resources. _____

2. I buy recycled paper and purchase biodegradable detergents and cleaning agents, or make my own cleaning products, whenever possible. _____

3. I recycle paper, plastic, and metals; purchase refillable containers when possible; and try to minimize the amount of paper and plastics that I use. _____

4. I try to wash my clothes only when they are dirty to reduce water consumption and the amount of detergents in our water sources. _____

5. I read articles and studies on environmental concerns to keep up to date on what I can do to help. _____

6. I donate clothing that is in good condition rather than throwing it away. _____

7. I turn down the heat and wear warmer clothes at home in winter and use the air conditioner only when necessary or at higher temperatures in summer. _____

8. When shopping for food, I purchase organic, locally grown, or in-season fruits and vegetables whenever possible. _____

9. I use both sides of the paper when taking class notes. _____

10. I minimize the amount of time that I run the faucet when I brush my teeth, shave, or shower. _____

Total score for this section: _____

Spiritual Health

Point Scale: 1 = Never, 2 = Rarely, 3 = Some of the time, 4 = Usually or always

1. I believe life is a precious gift that should be nurtured. _____
2. I take time to enjoy nature and the beauty around me. _____
3. I take time alone to think about what's important in life—who I am, what I value, where I fit in, and where I'm going. _____
4. I have faith in a greater power, be it a supreme being, nature, or the connectedness of all living things. _____
5. I engage in acts of caring and goodwill without expecting something in return. _____
6. I sympathize/empathize with those who are suffering and try to help them through difficult times. _____
7. I look forward to each day as an opportunity for further growth and challenge. _____
8. I work for peace in my interpersonal relationships, in my community, and in the world at large. _____
9. I have a great love and respect for all living things and regard all living creatures as important links in a vital chain. _____
10. I go for the gusto and experience life to the fullest. _____

Total score for this section: _____

Intellectual Health

Point Scale: 1 = Never, 2 = Rarely, 3 = Some of the time, 4 = Usually or always

1. I carefully consider my options and possible consequences as I make choices in life. _____
2. I learn from my mistakes and try to act differently the next time. _____
3. I follow directions or recommended guidelines, avoid risks, and act in ways likely to keep myself and others safe. _____
4. I consider myself a wise health consumer and check reliable information sources before making decisions. _____
5. I am alert and ready to respond to life's challenges in ways that reflect thought and sound judgment. _____
6. I have at least one hobby, learning activity, or personal growth activity that I make time for each week. _____
7. I actively learn all I can about products and services before making decisions. _____
8. I manage my time rather than let time manage me. _____
9. My friends and family trust my judgment. _____
10. I think about my self-talk (the things I tell myself) and then examine the evidence to see if my perceptions and feelings are sound. _____

Total score for this section: _____

Personal Health Promotion/Disease Prevention

Although each of the six dimensions of health are important, there are some factors that don't readily fit in one dimension. As college students, you face some unique risks that others may not have. For this reason, we have added a section to this self-assessment that focuses on personal health promotion and disease prevention. Answer these questions and add your results to the Personal Checklist in the following section.

Point Scale: 1 = Never, 2 = Rarely, 3 = Some of the time, 4 = Usually or always

1. I know the warning signs of common sexually transmitted infections, such as genital warts (HPV), chlamydia, and herpes, and read new information about these diseases as a way of protecting myself. _____
2. If I were to be sexually active, I would use protection such as latex condoms, dental dams, and other means of reducing my risk of sexually transmitted infections. _____

3. I can have a good time at parties or during happy hours without excessive drinking. ____

4. When I have more than 1 or 2 drinks, I ask someone who is not drinking to drive my friends and me home. ____

5. I am careful to use the appropriate safety equipment and precautions whenever I participate in a physical activity that could potentially cause bodily harm. ____

6. When I feel that I am getting sick, I slow down and take time to take care of myself so that I get better. ____

7. If I were to get a tattoo or piercing, I would go to a reputable person who follows strict standards of sterilization and precautions against blood-borne disease transmission. ____

8. I apply sunscreen, use products that contain a high SPF rating, and/or wear a hat and sunglasses whenever I engage in outdoor activities. ____

9. I am careful not to mix alcohol or other drugs with prescription and over-the-counter drugs. ____

10. I practice monthly breast/testicle self-examinations. ____

Total score for this section: ____

Personal Checklist

Now, total your scores in each of the health dimensions and compare them to what would be considered optimal scores. Which areas do you need to work on? How does your score compare with how you rated yourself in the first part of this chapter?

	Ideal Score	Your Score
Physical Health	40	____
Social Health	40	____
Emotional Health	40	____
Environmental Health	40	____
Spiritual Health	40	____
Intellectual Health	40	____
Personal Health Promotion	40	____
Disease Prevention	40	____

What Your Scores in Each Category Mean

Scores of 35–40: Your answers show that you are aware of the importance of these behaviors in your overall health. More importantly, you are putting your knowledge to work by practicing good health habits that should reduce your overall risks. Although you received a very high score on this part of the test, you may want to consider areas where your scores could be improved for your behavior change project.

Scores of 30–34: Your health practices in these areas are very good, but there is room for improvement. Look again at the items in which you scored 1 or 2 points. What changes could you make to improve your score? Even a small change in behavior can help you achieve better health.

Scores of 20–29: Your health risks are showing! Find information about the risks you are facing and why it is important to change these behaviors. Perhaps you need help in deciding how to make the changes you desire. Assistance is available from this book, your professor(s), and student health services at your school.

Scores below 20: You may be taking unnecessary risks with your health. Perhaps you are not aware of the risks and what to do about them. Identify each risk area and make a mental note as you read the associated chapter in your textbook. Whenever possible, seek additional resources, either on your campus or though your local community health resources, and make a serious commitment to behavior change. If any area is causing you to be less than functional in your class work or personal life, seek professional help.

In the sections that follow, you will find the information you need to help you improve your scores and your health. Remember that these scores are only indicators, not diagnostic tools.

Personalizing the Six Dimensions of Health

While you have already evaluated how healthy you are in the six dimensions of health, it is also important to understand how you feel about them. Use the following worksheet to personalize the six dimensions of health. For each component, write about an experience in which you demonstrated (or saw someone else demonstrate) a healthy attitude or activity. If you cannot remember or think of one, plan how you will demonstrate it in the future. These examples can be as varied in nature as working in a soup kitchen or planning to recycle on a regular basis.

Physical Health

_____

_____

_____

_____

How did this make you feel?

_____

_____

_____

Social Health

_____

_____

_____

_____

How did this make you feel?

_____

_____

_____

Emotional Health

_____

_____

_____

How did this make you feel?

_____

_____

Environmental Health

_____

_____

_____

How did this make you feel?

_____

_____

Spiritual Health

_____

_____

_____

How did this make you feel?

_____

_____

Intellectual Health

_____

_____

_____

_____

How did this make you feel?

_____

_____

_____

2 Plan Change

In order to successfully change a behavior, you must first begin by planning the steps you will need to make to create that change. This chapter will take you through all the steps necessary for beginning a behavior change.

ARE YOU READY?

In this section, you will continue to plan for your behavior change by reviewing the common target behaviors that most students plan to change and identifying your own targets. You will also have the chance to identify any addictive behaviors and begin monitoring your behavior. Are you ready?

Common Target Behaviors

Eight common target behaviors are examined below. If you think you are at risk for one or more of these behaviors, it is important to start a behavior change program.

Stress Management

Stress management is one of the most important behaviors in promoting good health. Proper stress reduction techniques and behavior modifications are important to establish in order to reduce your risk of disease and accidents. In this section, you will be able to assess the impact of stress on your life by answering the following questions.

DIRECTIONS: The purpose of this stress index questionnaire is to increase your awareness of the impact of stress on your life. Choose *Yes* or *No* for each of the stress index questions.

Yes   No   1. I have frequent arguments.

Yes   No   2. I often get upset at work.

Yes   No   3. I often have neck and/or shoulder pains due to anxiety or stress.

Yes   No   4. I often get upset when I stand in long lines.

Yes   No   5. I often get angry when I listen to the news or read the newspaper.

Yes   No   6. I worry about having a sufficient amount of money for my needs.

Yes   No   7. I often get upset when driving.

Yes   No   8. At the end of a work day, I often feel stress-related fatigue.

Yes   No   9. I have at least one constant source of stress/anxiety in my life (e.g., conflict with boss, neighbor, parents, etc.).

Yes   No   10. I often have stress-related headaches.

Yes   No   11. I do not practice stress management techniques.

Yes   No   12. I rarely take time for myself.

Yes   No   13. I have difficulty in keeping my feelings of anger and hostility under control.

Yes   No   14. I have difficulty in managing time wisely.

Yes   No   15. I often have difficulty sleeping.

Yes   No   16. I am generally in a hurry.

Yes   No   17. I usually feel that there is not enough time in the day to accomplish what I need to do.

Yes   No   18. I often feel that I am being mistreated by friends or associates.

Yes   No   19. I do not regularly perform physical activity.

Yes   No   20. I rarely get 7 to 8 hours of sleep per night.

EVALUATION

If you answered *Yes* to any of the questions, you might need to use some stress management techniques. Add your *Yes* answers and use the following scale to evaluate the level of stress in your life. If you're having difficulty handling the stress in your life, the worksheets in this log book will help you develop a plan to better manage it.

NUMBER OF *YES* ANSWERS

6–20   High stress
3–5   Average stress
0–2   Low stress

Tobacco Use

DATE ____

DIRECTIONS: Answer the following questions *True* or *False* to test your knowledge of the dangers of smoking.

T   F   1. Smoking increases your risk of lung cancer and heart disease.

T   F   2. Smoking is the most common avoidable cause of death.

T   F   3. Heavy smokers are 15–25 times more likely to die of cancer than nonsmokers.

T   F   4. Smoking soothes the throat and lungs by relaxing the cilia.

T   F   5. Smoking causes an increased risk of oral, pancreatic, and bladder cancer.

T   F   6. The average life expectancy for a chronic smoker is 7 years shorter than for a nonsmoker.

T   F   7. Smoking a pipe is less harmful than smoking cigarettes.

T   F   8. Pipes, cigarettes, and smokeless tobacco increase your risk of oral cancer.

T   F   9. Secondhand smoke is carcinogenic (cancer causing).

T   F   10. Chewing tobacco is harmless because there is no smoke to get into your lungs.

EVALUATION

Questions 4, 7, and 10 are *False*; all of the others are *True*. If you smoke or use tobacco, you are at risk for a number of health complications.

Sexual Health Awareness

This questionnaire is intended to get you thinking about your sexual health and is in no way a definitive evaluation of your risk of sexually transmitted infections (STIs). It is *always* a good idea to get tested before and after engaging in sexual activity with a new partner. STIs are generally spread through sexual contact but can also be contracted through shared needles or blood. There is no cure for HIV or herpes, and although treatment methods exist for many other STIs, prevention is always the best approach.

DATE ____

DIRECTIONS: For each of the following questions, please indicate the point value of each answer as it applies to you.

1. How often do you have sex? ____

   Never (0 points)
   Monthly or less (1 point)
   2–4 times a month (2 points)
   2–3 times a week (3 points)
   4 or more times a week (4 points)

2. When you have sex, how often do you use a condom or other form of barrier protection? ____

   Always/I don't have sex (0 points)
   Most of the time—4 out of 5 times (1 point)
   Sometimes—3 out of 5 times (2 points)
   Occasionally—1 or 2 out of 5 times (3 points)
   Never (4 points)

3. How often do you engage in oral sexual activity with a partner when either of you have cuts or sores on the mouth or genital tissues? ____

   Never/I don't have sex (0 points)
   Occasionally—1 or 2 out of 5 times (1 point)
   Sometimes—3 out of 5 times (2 points)
   Most of the time—4 out of 5 times (3 points)
   Frequently—4 out of 5 times (4 points)

4. In the past year, how many sexual partners have you had? ____

   None (0 points)
   One (1 point)
   Two to three (2 points)
   Four to five (3 points)
   Six or more (4 points)

5. In the past month, how often do you feel that your ability to make decisions about sex was compromised by substance use? ____

   Never/I don't have sex (0 points)
   Occasionally—1 out of 5 times (1 point)
   Sometimes—2 out of 5 times (2 points)
   Most of the time—3 out of 5 times (3 points)
   Frequently—4 out of 5 times (4 points)

PLAN CHANGE

6. When engaging in anal sex, do you take the appropriate precautions to minimize the risk of tears and infections? (Using lubricant, using a condom, changing condoms for anal and vaginal penetration, starting slowly, etc.) _____

Always/I don't have anal sex (0 points)

Most of the time—4 out of 5 times (1 point)

Sometimes—3 out of 5 times (2 points)

Occasionally—2 out of 5 times (3 points)

Never/Rarely (4 points)

7. When you have sex, how often do you and your partner use lubricant? _____

Always/I don't have sex (0 points)

Most of the time—4 out of 5 times (1 point)

Sometimes—3 out of 5 times (2 points)

Occasionally—2 out of 5 times (3 points)

Never/Rarely (4 points)

8. If you have a concern about your sexual health, do you ask your health care provider? _____

Yes, always (0 points)

Sometimes, but not always (1 point)

No, I usually don't (2 points)

9. Are you comfortable discussing sexual concerns and/or desires with a prospective partner? _____

Yes, always (0 points)

Sometimes, but not always (1 point)

No, I'm really not (2 points)

10. Before beginning sexual activities with a new partner, do you ask if he or she has any STIs? _____

Yes, always/don't have sex (0 points)

Sometimes, but not always (1 point)

No, I usually don't (2 points)

EVALUATION

Now, add up your answers. Total score: _____

If you feel you are not taking care of your sexual health, you should begin practicing safe sex and try to avoid alcohol, drugs, or other substances that may promote unsafe behavior. Visit a doctor or other health care provider for STI testing and information on ways to protect yourself.

Scores below 7: Based on your responses, it looks like you are in control of your sexual health and are taking steps to stay safe. Only you can really know if you are at risk for an STI, so if you feel that you might be at risk, it would be a good idea to get tested.

Scores between 8 and 10: Your current sexual practices are probably risky for your health. Try taking steps to change your behavior now, get tested, and make some positive changes for your (and your partners') health and safety.

Scores above 10: You are currently at a very high risk for getting an STI and passing it on to other partners. It would be a good idea to make an appointment with your health care provider to get tested. Look back at how you answered each question and identify some changes you can make to reduce your risk.

Cancer Prevention

Cancer is the second leading cause of death in the United States, and lifestyle habits such as smoking, eating high-fat diets, drinking excessively, and sunbathing are all contributors to an increased risk of cancer.

DATE ____

DIRECTIONS: Answer the following questions *Yes* or *No* to determine your risk.

Yes No   1. Do you consume a high-fat diet (i.e., >30 percent total calorie intake)?

Yes No   2. Is your diet low in fiber?

Yes No   3. Do you consume an excessive amount of alcohol?

Yes No   4. Do you regularly eat smoked foods?

Yes No   5. Are you exposed to environmental carcinogens (cancer-causing agents)?

Yes No   6. Do you use tobacco products or breathe secondhand smoke?

Yes No   7. Are you obese?

Yes No   8. Do you have a family history of cancer?

Yes No   9. Is your skin regularly exposed to excessive sunlight?

Yes No 10. Do you have a fair complexion?

EVALUATION

Answering *Yes* to any of the questions means that you should modify your lifestyle to reduce your risk of cancer. Reduce your risk of cancer by maintaining a healthy diet, exercising regularly, avoiding carcinogens, and limiting excess exposure to the sun. For further information, see your text.

Healthy Eating

Are you getting the most out of your food? With so many food choices in the dining hall and grocery store, it can be hard to tell if you are making nutritious decisions.

DATE ____

DIRECTIONS: Answer the following questions *Yes* or *No* to determine if you are eating right.

Yes No   1. Do you eat breakfast?

Yes No   2. Are grains the main food choice at all or most of your meals?

Yes No   3. Do you take a multivitamin or any type of food supplement?

Yes No   4. Do you carry a healthy snack for when you get hungry?

Yes No   5. Do you drink more water than soda?

Yes No   6. Do you often forget to eat vegetables?

Yes No   7. Do you typically eat fewer than three pieces of fruit daily?

PLAN CHANGE

Yes   No   8. Do you consume less than the daily recommended amount of dairy? (1 cup of milk or 1.5 oz of cheese)

Yes   No   9. Do you always count the calories in every food item you consume?

Yes   No   10. Are you worried that you are not eating as well as you should?

EVALUATION

If you answered *No* to questions 1–5 and *Yes* to questions 6–10, you should begin taking steps to adopt healthier eating habits.

Getting and Staying Fit

We often have an unrealistic perception of how much we actively move, yet maintaining your physical fitness now is an important way to avoid health problems later.

DATE ____

DIRECTIONS: Answer *Yes* or *No* to the following questions to begin evaluating your fitness level.

Yes   No   1. When you walk up a flight of stairs, do you have to catch your breath at the top?

Yes   No   2. Do you have difficulty touching your toes while keeping your knees straight?

Yes   No   3. Are you in the habit of taking the elevator more than the stairs?

Yes   No   4. Do you make up excuses to avoid exercising?

Yes   No   5. Do you work out too hard and injure yourself?

Yes   No   6. Is your schedule set up in a way that gives you regular periods of exercise?

Yes   No   7. Do you make an effort to walk to places that are easily reachable by foot?

Yes   No   8. Do you try to find new and interesting fitness programs/classes to try?

Yes   No   9. Can you jog or run continuously for 20 minutes?

Yes   No   10. Do you engage in some sort of physical activity for 30 minutes every day?

EVALUATION

If you answered *Yes* to questions 1–5 and *No* to questions 6–10, you should begin taking steps to change your fitness habits. If you are not as physically active as you would like, use this log book to develop strategies and goals for modifying your behavior. Be sure to visit your primary care physician for a general check-up and to address any injuries that you might have. You can also check with the athletic department at your school to see if there is a physical/athletic trainer who can help you set up a personalized fitness program.

Alcohol Use

The consumption of alcoholic drinks is a part of many events on most college campuses. Research shows that very low consumption of some types of alcohol can be beneficial, but too much can be dangerous for your health. Do you need to change your drinking habits? The following evaluation will help you decide.

DATE ____

DIRECTIONS: For each of the following questions, please indicate the point value of each answer as it applies to you.

1. How often do you have a drink containing alcohol? _____

   Never (0 points)
   Monthly or less (1 point)
   2–4 times a month (2 points)
   2–3 times a week (3 points)
   4 or more times a week (4 points)

2. How many alcoholic drinks do you have on a typical day when you are drinking? _____

   1 or 2 (0 points)
   3 or 4 (1 point)
   5 or 6 (2 points)
   7 to 9 (3 points)
   10 or more (4 points)

3. How often do you have six drinks or more on one occasion? _____

   Never (0 points)
   Less than monthly (1 point)
   Monthly (2 points)
   Weekly (3 points)
   Daily or almost daily (4 points)

4. How often during the last year have you been unable to stop drinking once you had started? _____

   Never (0 points)
   Less than monthly (1 point)
   Monthly (2 points)
   Weekly (3 points)
   Daily or almost daily (4 points)

5. How often during the last year have you failed to do what was normally expected from you because of drinking? _____

   Never (0 points)
   Less than monthly (1 point)
   Monthly (2 points)
   Weekly (3 points)
   Daily or almost daily (4 points)

6. How often during the last year have you needed a first drink in the morning to get yourself going after a heavy drinking session? _____

   Never (0 points)

   Less than monthly (1 point)

   Monthly (2 points)

   Weekly (3 points)

   Daily or almost daily (4 points)

7. How often during the last year have you had a feeling of guilt or remorse after drinking? _____

   Never (0 points)

   Less than monthly (1 point)

   Monthly (2 points)

   Weekly (3 points)

   Daily or almost daily (4 points)

8. How often during the last year have you been unable to remember what happened the night before because you had been drinking? _____

   Never (0 points)

   Less than monthly (1 point)

   Monthly (2 points)

   Weekly (3 points)

   Daily or almost daily (4 points)

9. Have you or someone else been injured as a result of your drinking? _____

   No (0 points)

   Yes, but not in the last year (1 point)

   Yes, during the last year (2 points)

10. Has a relative, friend, or doctor or other health worker been concerned about your drinking or suggested that you cut down? _____

   No (0 points)

   Yes, but not in the last year (1 point)

   Yes, during the last year (2 points)

EVALUATION

Now, add up your answers. Total score: _____

Scores below 5: Based on your responses to this questionnaire, you are in control of your drinking behaviors and do a good job consuming alcohol responsibly and in moderation.

Scores between 6 and 8: Your alcohol consumption is possibly risky for your health. Try taking steps to change your drinking behavior and make some positive changes for your health and safety.

Scores above 8: Your drinking patterns are putting you at high risk for illness, unsafe sexual situations, and alcohol-related injuries and may even affect your academic performance. Look back at how you answered each question, and identify some changes you can make to reduce your risk.

Source: Adapted from the AUDIT Manual, box 4, p. 17, World Health Organization, Division of Mental Health and Prevention of Substance Abuse. http://whqlibdoc.who.int/hq/2001/WHO_MSD_MSB_01.6a.pdf. Copyright (C) 2001 World Health Organization.

Adequate Sleep

Everyone needs sleep, but are you getting as much as you need? Most college students are not getting enough quality sleep, which makes their daytime activities, like schoolwork, class participation, and extracurricular activities, suffer.

DATE _____

DIRECTIONS: Answer *Yes* or *No* to the following questions to determine if you are getting enough sleep.

Yes   No   1. Do you avoid the use of caffeine, alcohol, or other substances after 8 p.m.?

Yes   No   2. Do you give yourself at least one hour to "unwind" before going to bed?

Yes   No   3. Do you have a comfortable bed and pillow?

Yes   No   4. Is the temperature in your room about 68°F when you sleep?

Yes   No   5. Do you have a regular sleep time and wake time?

Yes   No   6. Do you get about 20 minutes of sunlight per day?

Yes   No   7. Do you get at least 7–8 hours of sleep per night?

Yes   No   8. Is the room darkened when you are sleeping?

Yes   No   9. Do you usually wake up in the morning feeling refreshed?

Yes   No   10. Do you sleep straight through the night without waking up multiple times?

EVALUATION

If you answered *No* to any of these questions, you are probably not getting the best sleep and should begin making changes to how you sleep. If you think your sleep is being compromised due to a medical problem, be sure to visit your primary care physician

Your Target Behaviors

DATE ____

DIRECTIONS: In the following spaces, list five behaviors that you want to change. They might be behaviors discussed earlier in this chapter or others specific to you. Examples of target behaviors include smoking, eating unhealthy foods, and not exercising regularly.

Target Behaviors:

1. _____
2. _____
3. _____
4. _____
5. _____

Choose the target behavior you feel the most strongly about changing, and use the following worksheets and logs to help you modify that behavior. Once you've succeeded in changing that behavior, choose another one to work on.

Understanding Your Target Behavior: Is It Addictive?

DATE ____

DIRECTIONS: To help you decide if your target behavior is addictive, answer the following questions, substituting your target behavior in the blanks.

Yes   No   1. Do you _____ alone?

Yes   No   2. Do you _____ on a regular basis?

Yes   No   3. When you are stressed, do you _____?

Yes   No   4. Do you crave _____ at any time of the day?

Yes   No   5. Are you influenced by others to _____?

Yes   No   6. Does your _____ impair your job performance or ability to engage in daily activities?

Yes   No   7. Does your _____ cause you to use poor judgment?

Yes   No   8. Do you lie to friends or family about how much or how often you _____?

Yes   No   9. Have you tried unsuccessfully to cut down on _____?

EVALUATION

If you answered *Yes* to any of these questions, you may be addicted. If this addiction affects your health (e.g., smoking) you should talk with a physician or other health care provider.

Understanding Your Target Behavior: What Are Its Health Effects?

To better understand the importance of your behavior change, it is important to recognize the harmful effects of your present target behavior and the positive effects of quitting that behavior.

Some negative health effects of my target behavior are:

1. _____
2. _____
3. _____
4. _____

Some positive health effects of changing my behavior will be:

1. _____
2. _____
3. _____
4. _____

Understanding Your Target Behavior: Monitoring Your Behavior

In order to better understand why and when you engage in your target behavior, use the following log to keep track of it for the next 3 days. Be sure to make a note of the events and feelings that were present when you engaged in your target behavior as they will create a better understanding of your motivations.

DIRECTIONS: Use this table to monitor your target behavior for at least 3 days.

Date	How long did it last? Intensity?	When did it occur?	Where did it occur?

What else were you doing?	Other influences?	Your thoughts and feelings about it?

SET GOALS, TIMELINES, AND REWARDS

In this section, you will begin to plan out the change you would like to make in your current behavior by setting goals, planning a timeline, and choosing your rewards. The worksheets that follow will help you create the structure for your behavior change project.

Goals

Whatever your target behavior is, there are several key points to remember when establishing goals.

1. Establish achievable goals.
2. Put goals in writing and place them where you can see them every day.
3. Establish both short- and long-term goals.
4. Establish goals that are measurable.
5. Set target dates for achieving goals.
6. After you achieve a goal, establish another achievable goal.
7. Reward yourself after achievement of a goal.

Timelines

When it comes to creating a timeline for your goals, it is always a good idea to make it *manageable*. The best timeline is one that requires you to reach out of your comfort zone. But don't make it discouraging! Track yourself with small goals every few weeks that lead up to the greater behavior change.

DIRECTIONS: Fill out the spaces below to assist you in setting your goals on a timeline.

Short-Term Goal #1: _____

Date to Achieve: _____

Short-Term Goal #2: _____

Date to Achieve: _____

Short-Term Goal #3: _____

Date to Achieve: _____

Short-Term Goal #4: _____

Date to Achieve: _____

Short-Term Goal #5: _____

Date to Achieve: _____

Short-Term Goal #6: _____

Date to Achieve: _____

Long-Term Goal: _____

Date to Achieve: _____

Don't forget to mark your short-term goals on a calendar or set up a reminder system so that you remember them!

Rewards

It is important to reward yourself for accomplishments and goals that you have met. Rewards should be things that you may not always get to do, but things that you enjoy doing. They should be relatively inexpensive and accessible, and they should not be anything that reinforces the behavior you are trying to change. Rewards for someone trying to lose weight might be shopping or taking a walk on the beach, rather then going out to eat or eating sweets.

DIRECTIONS: Fill out the spaces below to assist you in setting your rewards.

Short-Term Goal #1: _____

Reward: _____

Short-Term Goal #2: _____

Reward: _____

Short-Term Goal #3: _____

Reward: _____

Short-Term Goal #4: _____

Reward: _____

Short-Term Goal #5: _____

Reward: _____

Short-Term Goal #6: _____

Reward: _____

Long-Term Goal: _____

Reward: _____

IDENTIFY OBSTACLES AND SOLUTIONS

After establishing your short-term and long-term goals for behavior change, you will find that there will be many distractions and challenges that may hinder your progress. In order to overcome these obstacles, you must develop strategies to counteract them.

For example, Susan has decided that she wants to lose weight. She has established a program for herself that includes eating healthy, proportionate meals every day, and exercising at least 5 days a week. Susan has been invited to a Super Bowl party that includes a big barbeque with lots of food, chips, sweets, and beer. She really wants to go to the party but does not want to break her weight loss program. What strategies can Susan use to overcome this obstacle?

Some suggestions for Susan might be to eat a healthy meal before the barbeque so that when she arrives she is not hungry and possibly not as tempted as if she arrived with an empty stomach. Susan might also bring a plate of vegetables and low-fat dip to share with the guests. If she is hungry, she should stick to the healthier snack that she brought or eat some of the other food in moderation. Susan might also want to socialize with guests in an area away from the food. After the party, she should reward herself for overcoming the temptations by engaging in an activity that she enjoys.

Examining Attitudes and Developing Strategies

Understanding your attitudes and feelings about your target behavior will help you better understand why you engage in that behavior and what might prevent you from changing it. This knowledge will allow you to create effective strategies to overcome obstacles.

DIRECTIONS: Fill in the blanks with the appropriate answers.

I engage in _____ because _____
  (target behavior)

_____

I am most tempted to _____ when _____
  (target behavior)

_____

I have not quit _____ because _____
  (target behavior)

_____

_____ is difficult for me because _____
  (behavior goal)

_____

_____

I feel that _____ would help me to achieve _____
  (strategy 1)   (behavior goal)

because _____

I feel that _____ would help me to achieve _____
  (strategy 2)   (behavior goal)

because _____

I feel that _____ would help me to achieve _____
  (strategy 3)   (behavior goal)

because _____

Once I achieve _____, I can stick to it by _____
  (behavior goal)   (maintenance strategy)

_____

COMMIT TO CHANGE

Now that you've completed all the steps to prepare for a behavior change, it is time to affirm your commitment to making a healthy change! In the following pages, you will be able to fill out a behavior change contract for a short, semester-long project and a contract that is designed for a lifetime behavior change. Both contracts come with examples for you to follow.

Behavior Change Contract

DIRECTIONS: Choose a see health behavior that you would like to change and fill out this behavior change contract (a sample on the next page). Sign the contract at the bottom to affirm your commitment to making a healthy change, and ask a friend to witness it.

My behavior change will be:

_____

My long-term goal for this behavior change is:

_____

These are three obstacles to change (things that I am currently doing or situations that contribute to this behavior or make it harder to change):

   1. _____

   2. _____

   3. _____

The strategies that I will use to overcome these obstacles are:

   1. _____

   2. _____

   3. _____

Resources I will use to help me change this behavior include:

A friend/partner/relative: _____

A school-based resource: _____

A community-based resource: _____

A book or reputable website: _____

In order to make my goal more attainable, I have devised these short-term goals.

_____	_____	_____
(short-term goal 1)	(target date)	(reward)
_____	_____	_____
(short-term goal 2)	(target date)	(reward)
_____	_____	_____
(short-term goal 3)	(target date)	(reward)

When I make the long-term behavior change described above, my reward will be:

_____ Target Date: _____

I intend to make the behavior change described above. I will use the strategies and rewards to achieve the goals that will contribute to a healthy behavior change.

Signed: _____   Witness: _____

Sample Behavior Change Contract

My behavior change will be:

To snack less on junk food and more on healthy foods

My long-term goal for this behavior change is:

Eat junk food snacks no more than once a week

These are three obstacles to change (things that I am currently doing or situations that contribute to this behavior or make it harder to change):

1. The grocery store is closed by the time I come home from school.

2. I get hungry between classes and the vending machines only carry candy bars.

3. It's easier to order pizza or other snacks than to make a snack at home.

The strategies that I will use to overcome these obstacles are:

1. I'll leave early for school once a week so I can stock up on healthy snacks in the morning.

2. I'll bring a piece of fruit or other healthy snack to eat between classes.

3. I'll learn some easy recipes for snacks to make at home.

Resources I will use to help me change this behavior include:

A friend/partner/relative: My roommates: I'll ask them to buy healthier snacks instead of chips when they do the shopping.

A school-based resource: The dining hall: I'll ask them to provide healthy foods we can take to eat between classes.

A community-based resource: The library: I'll check out some cookbooks to find easy snack ideas.

A book or reputable website: The USDA nutrient database: I'll use this site to make sure the foods I select are healthy choices.

In order to make my goal more attainable, I have devised these short-term goals.

Eat a healthy snack 3 times per week	9/15	New book
(short-term goal 1)	(target date)	(reward)
Learn to make a healthy snack	10/15	Concert ticket
(short-term goal 2)	(target date)	(reward)
Eat a healthy snack 5 times per week	11/15	New shoes
(short-term goal 3)	(target date)	(reward)

When I make the long-term behavior change described above, my reward will be:

Ski lift tickets for winter break   Target Date: 12/15

I intend to make the behavior change described above. I will use the strategies and rewards to achieve the goals that will contribute to a healthy behavior change.

Signed: Elizabeth King   Witness: Susan Bauer

Lifelong Behavior Change Contract

Behavior change is a process that continues for a lifetime. The strategies that you begin to follow now can contribute to healthy benefits far into the future. Choose a change that will have long-term positive effects, then complete the contract and put your intentions into action (see a sample filled-in contract on the next page). Sign the contract at the bottom to affirm your commitment to making a healthy change, and ask a friend to witness it.

My behavior change will be:

_____

My long-term goal for this behavior change is:

_____

These are three obstacles to change (things that I am currently doing or situations that contribute to this behavior or make it harder to change):

1. _____
2. _____
3. _____

The strategies that I will use to overcome these obstacles are:

1. _____
2. _____
3. _____

Resources I will use to help me change this behavior include:

A friend/partner/relative: _____

A school-based resource: _____

A community-based resource: _____

A book or reputable website:_____

In order to make my goal more attainable, I have devised these short-term goals.

_____	_____	_____
(short-term goal 1)	(target date)	(reward)
_____	_____	_____
(short-term goal 2)	(target date)	(reward)
_____	_____	_____
(short-term goal 3)	(target date)	(reward)

When I make the long-term behavior change described above, my reward will be:

_____ Target Date: _____

I intend to make the behavior change described above. I will use the strategies and rewards to achieve the goals that will contribute to a healthy behavior change.

Signed: _____   Witness: _____

Sample Lifelong Behavior Change Contract

My behavior change will be:

To incorporate exercise into my daily life

My long-term goal for this behavior change is:

To maintain a healthy weight and feel fit

These are three obstacles to change (things that I am currently doing or situations that contribute to this behavior or make it harder to change):

1. I get bored doing the same exercise all of the time.

2. I find myself watching TV I don't even enjoy and then not having time to exercise.

3. I'm afraid I'll injure myself doing new activities.

The strategies that I will use to overcome these obstacles are:

1. I'll learn several activities so that I have variety in my exercise program.

2. I'll give myself a set number of "TV hours" and use the extra time for exercise.

3. I'll get a complete check-up with my physician before I start a new exercise program.

Resources I will use to help me change this behavior include:

A friend/partner/relative: I'll ask friends to exercise with me so I stay motivated and don't get bored.

A school-based resource: I'll find out what types of activities are offered by the PE department.

A community-based resource: I'll join a local club that does the activity I enjoy most.

A book or reputable website: I'll track my progress in the Fitness section of my Log Book and Wellness Journal.

In order to make my goal more attainable, I have devised these short-term goals.

Walk to school 3 times a week	3 months from today	dinner out at my favorite restaurant
(short-term goal 1)	(target date)	(reward)
Learn a new fitness activity	6 months from today	new outfit
(short-term goal 2)	(target date)	(reward)
Participate in the local 10k walk/run	1 year from today	weekend vacation
(short-term goal 3)	(target date)	(reward)

When I make the long-term behavior change described above, my reward will be:

vacation trip   Target Date: 2 years from now

I intend to make the behavior change described above. I will use the strategies and rewards to achieve the goals that will contribute to a healthy behavior change.

Signed: Barry Snow   Witness: Rob Santiago

3 Implement Change

While this workbook provides a general log for goals of your choice, in this chapter we have also provided logs specifically designed for changes in diet, weight management, and particular fitness goals.

GOAL LOG

Use this log to track your progress. If you have set daily goals, use the log daily; if you have set weekly goals, use the log weekly. If you need inspiration, there are sample goal logs provided after the blank logs.

Target Behavior	Date	Goal	Goal Achieved?	What Happened?	New Strategy/ New Goal

Target Behavior	Date	Goal	Goal Achieved?	What Happened?	New Strategy/ New Goal

Target Behavior	Date	Goal	Goal Achieved?	What Happened?	New Strategy/ New Goal

Target Behavior	Date	Goal	Goal Achieved?	What Happened?	New Strategy/ New Goal

Target Behavior	Date	Goal	Goal Achieved?	What Happened?	New Strategy/ New Goal

Target Behavior	Date	Goal	Goal Achieved?	What Happened?	New Strategy/ New Goal

Sample Goal Logs

While we cannot provide you with sample goal logs for every behavior, the samples that follow cover some of the more common behaviors. Use them to help get started on your own!

Sample Stress Management Goal Log

Target Behavior	Date	Goal	Goal Achieved?	What Happened?	New Strategy/ New Goal
Excessive stress	12/1–12/8	Study for test w/o stressing out	Yes	When I felt stressed I took a 10 min jog & then went back to studying	Next time I get stressed studying I'll take a 5 min jog

Sample Tobacco Use Goal Log

Target Behavior	Date	Goal	Goal Achieved?	What Happened?	New Strategy/ New Goal
Smoking	3/7–3/21	Cut down to ½ pack per week by 3/21	No	Smoked a lot of cigarettes at a party	Next time I'm at a party I'll try to avoid being around people who smoke

Sample Sexual Health Awareness Goal Log

Target Behavior	Date	Goal	Goal Achieved?	What Happened?	New Strategy/ New Goal
Poor sexual decision-making	10/8	Use condoms every time I have sex	Yes	Had to borrow a condom from a friend when I wanted to have sex	Next time I'll be prepared and buy my own condoms

Sample Cancer Prevention Goal Log

Target Behavior	Date	Goal	Goal Achieved?	What Happened?	New Strategy/ New Goal
Sunbathing w/o sunscreen	6/17	Use at least SPF 15 when outdoors; reapply regularly	No	Forgot to bring sunscreen to the beach	Now I'll keep the sunscreen in my car so that I'll have it when I drive to the ocean

Sample Healthy Eating Goal Log

Target Behavior	Date	Goal	Goal Achieved?	What Happened?	New Strategy/ New Goal
Unhealthy eating	5/9	Eat more healthy snacks	Yes	Remembered to grab an apple from the dining hall after lunch for a snack later	Next time I'll prepare something healthy to snack on

Sample Getting and Staying Fit Goal Log

Target Behavior	Date	Goal	Goal Achieved?	What Happened?	New Strategy/ New Goal
Avoiding exercise	2/6–2/13	Work out 3 times a week for an hour each time	No	Worked out twice but friends were watching a movie when I attempted to go a third time so I skipped to watch with them	Next time I'll set up specific days and times to work out

Sample Alcohol Use Goal Log

Target Behavior	Date	Goal	Goal Achieved?	What Happened?	New Strategy/ New Goal
Drinking too much	10/5–10/12	Limit the number of drinks I have at a time to less than 3	Yes	Drank slowly to stretch the drinks out over the evening	Next time I'll drink water between drinks

Sample Adequate Sleep Goal Log

Target Behavior	Date	Goal	Goal Achieved?	What Happened?	New Strategy/ New Goal
Staying up late	8/11	Get better sleep	No	Couldn't fall asleep and ended up watching TV late	Next time I'll create a "calming down" period before I go to bed

BEHAVIOR CHANGE JOURNAL ENTRIES

As you complete your behavior change project, use this journal section to record your thoughts and feelings about your progress. We've included some project-specific prompts for you to get started along with a set of blank pages for more open-ended journaling.

Day One of Your Behavior Change Project

Complete this journal response on the first day or two of your behavior change project.

Which behavior are you trying to change and why? Do you think it will be easy or difficult to change your behavior? Right now, how do you feel about your behavior change project? Are you excited, ambivalent, or nervous? What do you think will be your greatest obstacle to changing your behavior?

NAME: _____ DATE: _____

_____

_____

_____

_____

_____

_____

_____

_____

_____

_____

_____

_____

_____

_____

_____

_____

_____

_____

_____

_____

_____

_____

Weeks 1–2 of Your Behavior Change Project

Complete this journal response by the end of the second week of your behavior change project.

Now that you've started trying to change your behavior, how do you feel about it? Has it been easier or harder to change than you expected? Why do you think that is? Have you achieved any goals or rewards yet? Have you encountered any obstacles? Which? If you've encountered an obstacle to changing your behavior, how will you avoid it in the future?

NAME: _____   DATE: _____

_____

_____

_____

_____

_____

_____

_____

_____

_____

_____

_____

_____

_____

_____

_____

_____

_____

IMPLEMENT CHANGE: JOURNALING

Middle of Your Behavior Change Project

Complete this journal response somewhere in the middle of your behavior change project.

How do you feel about your behavior change now that you are in the middle of the project? Has it become any easier or harder to change? Why do you think that is? Have you achieved any goals or rewards yet? Have you encountered any obstacles? Which? If you've encountered an obstacle to changing your behavior, how will you avoid it in the future?

NAME: _____   DATE: _____

_____

_____

_____

_____

_____

_____

_____

_____

_____

_____

_____

_____

_____

_____

_____

_____

_____

_____

_____

_____

End of Your Behavior Change Project

Complete this journal response at the end of your behavior change project.

Congratulations, you've completed your behavior change project! Look back over your journal entries; how did it go? Was it easy for you to change your behavior, or did you have a harder time than you expected? Will you continue to maintain your behavior change? How will you accomplish this and why? Was this project helpful to you?

NAME: _____   DATE: _____

_____

_____

_____

_____

_____

_____

_____

_____

_____

_____

_____

_____

_____

_____

_____

_____

_____

_____

_____

_____

_____

_____

Stress Management

How are you feeling today? Are you more or less stressed than you were yesterday? Use these journal pages to brainstorm activities that might help you manage your stress in the future. You can also use these pages to list the things that make you stressed and how you are going to change their effect on your health.

NAME: _____   DATE: _____

_____

_____

_____

_____

_____

_____

_____

_____

_____

_____

_____

_____

_____

_____

_____

_____

_____

_____

_____

_____

Tobacco Use

How does using tobacco affect your life? Do you find that there are certain times during the day when you use it? On these journal pages, list when the times and events during which you most commonly found yourself using or needing tobacco during the past week. Then brainstorm how you can change any of these to reduce your tobacco consumption.

NAME: _____   DATE: _____

_____

_____

_____

_____

_____

_____

_____

_____

_____

_____

_____

_____

_____

_____

_____

_____

_____

_____

_____

_____

IMPLEMENT CHANGE: JOURNALING

_____

_____

_____

_____

_____

_____

_____

_____

_____

_____

_____

_____

_____

_____

_____

_____

_____

_____

_____

_____

_____

_____

_____

Sexual Health Awareness

Practicing safe sex is only a small component of taking care of your sexual health. What are other ways that you can improve your sexual health? Use the following journal pages to brainstorm ways that you can improve your sexual health. These can range from sharing a fantasy with your partner, to taking a class, to becoming more comfortable with your sexual self.

NAME: _____　　DATE: _____

_____

_____

_____

_____

_____

_____

_____

_____

_____

_____

_____

_____

_____

_____

_____

_____

_____

_____

_____

_____

_____

IMPLEMENT CHANGE: JOURNALING

Cancer Prevention

What types of cancers do you think you and your friends are at greatest risk for right now? What are you doing to reduce your risk? Use these journal pages to list the different types of cancers that you feel you are at greatest risk for right now and ways that you can reduce that risk.

NAME: _____   DATE: _____

_____

_____

_____

_____

_____

_____

_____

_____

_____

_____

_____

_____

_____

_____

_____

_____

_____

_____

_____

_____

_____

_____

_____

IMPLEMENT CHANGE: JOURNALING

Healthy Eating

What are the reasons behind why you eat what you eat? Do you have control over your meal choices, or are you a captive of the dining hall menu? Use these journal pages to write about your feelings regarding your food choices and brainstorm ways to improve your eating habits. If you are already eating well, write about the choices you had to make to get you to this point.

NAME: _____   DATE: _____

_____

_____

_____

_____

_____

_____

_____

_____

_____

_____

_____

_____

_____

_____

_____

_____

_____

Managing Your Weight

How do you feel about your current weight? Are you happy with how you look, or do you find yourself regularly worrying about that extra pound or two? While maintaining a healthy weight is important to your overall health, it is equally important to be body positive and comfortable with how you are built. Use these journal pages to write down some things that you like about yourself and why.

NAME: _____   DATE: _____

_____

_____

_____

_____

_____

_____

_____

_____

_____

_____

_____

_____

_____

_____

_____

_____

_____

_____

_____

Getting and Staying Fit

How does your definition of physical fitness compare with the definition presented in your health class? Which components are the most motivating to you to start or continue a fitness program? Use these journal pages to write about what physical fitness means to you. If you are just beginning a fitness program, you can also use these pages to write out a detailed fitness plan.

NAME: _____   DATE: _____

_____

_____

_____

_____

_____

_____

_____

_____

_____

_____

_____

_____

_____

_____

_____

_____

_____

_____

_____

_____

Alcohol Use

Do you remember your first alcoholic drink? How did you feel about it? Have your drinking habits changed any since then? Use these journal pages to write about your current drinking habits and how they might be affecting you in a positive or negative way.

NAME: _____   DATE: _____

_____

_____

_____

_____

_____

_____

_____

_____

_____

_____

_____

_____

_____

_____

_____

_____

_____

_____

_____

_____

_____

_____

_____

Adequate Sleep

How did you sleep last night? Use these journal pages as a sleep diary. Be sure to record approximately when you fell asleep, when you woke up in the morning, if you woke up multiple times in the night, and how you felt in the morning. Mention any dreams you had. Do you see any patterns in how you sleep?

NAME: _____   DATE: _____

_____

_____

_____

_____

_____

_____

_____

_____

_____

_____

_____

_____

_____

_____

_____

_____

_____

_____

_____

_____

_____

Open Journaling

The following pages are intentionally left blank for you to journal your behavior change experience without any prompts. Use this section in whatever way you feel is most helpful to you!

IMPROVING NUTRITION

Nutrition and weight management are critical aspects of a healthy lifestyle. A change in your lifestyle that emphasizes proper nutrition and weight management can lower your risk of disease and improve your health and well-being. This section will help you get started.

MyPlate

For fitness and wellness, nutrition is one of the most important considerations. Nutrients provide energy and the essential molecules necessary for shaping and operating the body's systems. The adage is true: "You are what you eat."

MyPlate (below) is a great place to begin planning a new diet.

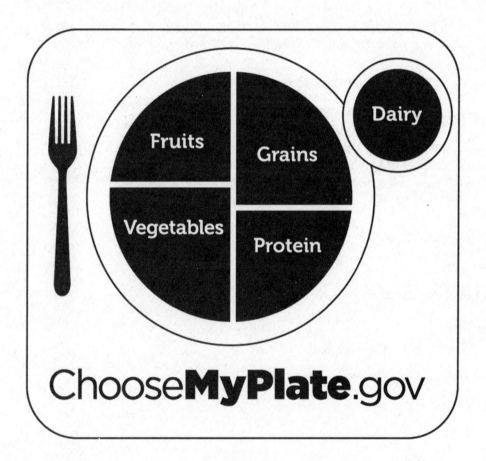

MyPlate is a food guidance system based on the *Dietary Guidelines for Americans, 2010*, replacing the previously used MyPyramid. Through the illustration of a familiar meal place setting, this new MyPlate icon is intended to remind you to eat healthfully. Visit www.ChooseMyPlate.gov to assess your current diet and physical activity levels and also access an interactive and personalized food plan. Tips are available on the website to help you make healthy changes in your current food choices and physical activity patterns.

Reflective of the *Dietary Guidelines for Americans, 2010*, MyPlate encourages you to eat for health through three general areas of recommendation:

1. Balance calories:
   - Enjoy your food, but eat less.
   - Avoid oversized portions.
2. Foods to increase:
   - Make half your plate fruits and vegetables.
   - Make at least half your grains whole.
   - Switch to fat-free or 1% milk.
3. Foods to reduce:
   - Compare sodium in foods like soup, bread, and frozen meals—and choose the foods with lower numbers.
   - Drink water instead of sugary drinks

The new MyPlate takes into consideration the dietary and caloric needs for a wide variety of individuals, such as pregnant or breastfeeding women, those trying to lose weight, and adults with different activity levels.

Source: U.S. Department of Agriculture, Center for Nutrition Policy and Promotion, 2011.

Portion Sizes

When figuring out your daily nutrient intake, you have to take into account *how much* you are eating. You may be confused by how much an ounce, a cup, or a "medium" apple is. The list below gives you a general idea of how to relate these measures to what's on your plate.

- 1 medium apple

  —the size of a baseball

- 1 teaspoon (5 ml)

  —the volume of your little finger

- 1 ounce (28 g)

  —1 slice of bread or cheese (sandwich size)

  —enough nuts to cover the palm of your hand

  —1/8 of a medium apple

- 2 ounces (56 g)

  —1/4 of a medium apple

  —1/2 cup of peanut butter

- 4 ounces (112 g)

  —1 fish filet

  —1 small orange

  —1 hamburger patty

- 1/2 cup (118 ml)

  —a handful of dried fruit

  —a water cooler cup

- 1 cup (236 ml)

  —about the volume of a baseball

  —volume of a standard light bulb

Diet Assessment

Use the following logs to record your daily dietary habits for 3 days (try to include weekdays and weekend days). The new MyPlate and USDA's recommended dietary allowance and intake values for different nutrients will help you determine where changes in your diet need to be made.

Notes to Diet Assessment

For detailed information on the nutritional content of your diet, you can enter the foods from your logs and assessments into the MyPyramidTracker at www.mypyramidtracker.gov or into your instructor's recommended diet analysis software. (The MyPyramidTracker has been updated to incorporate the new MyPlate recommendations, even though the name of the tracker has not changed.)

* Your daily kcal requirement is determined by your daily caloric expenditure (see page 82). You can create a nutritional calorie deficit to lose weight, but it should be no more than 250 kcal/day.

† Your daily protein intake should be _____ × 0.36 g/lb = _____ g.

                      (body weight in lbs)

‡ Calcium: Males and females 9–18 years old need 1300 mg, 19–50 years old need 1000 mg, and 51 and older need 1200 mg.

§ Iron: Males 9–13 years old and 19 and older need 8 mg, 14–18 years old need 11 mg. Females 9–13 years old and 51 and older need 8 mg, 14–18 years old need 15 mg, 19–50 years old need 18 mg, pregnant (any age) need 27 mg, and lactating need 9 mg if over 19 years old and 10 mg if under.

DAY ONE Food	Vegetable Servings	Breads and Cereals Servings	Fruit Servings	Dairy Servings	Meats and Protein Servings	Calories (kcals)	Protein (gm)	Carbohydrate (g)	Fiber (g)	Fat (g)	Total Fat % (kcal)	Saturated Fat (g)	Cholestorol (mg)	Sodium (mg)	Vitamin A (ug)	Vitamin C (mg)	Calcium (mg)	Iron (mg)
TOTALS																		
Recommendations	3–5	6–11	2–4	2–3	2–3	See note *	See note †	>58% of diet	30% of diet	<30% of diet	From food label	<10% of diet	<300 mg	3000 mg	700–900 ug	65–90 mg	See note ‡	See note §

DAY TWO Food	Vegetable Servings	Breads and Cereals Servings	Fruit Servings	Dairy Servings	Meats and Protein Servings	Calories (kcals)	Protein (gm)	Carbohydrate (g)	Fiber (g)	Fat (g)	Total Fat % (kcal)	Saturated Fat (g)	Cholestorol (mg)	Sodium (mg)	Vitamin A (ug)	Vitamin C (mg)	Calcium (mg)	Iron (mg)
TOTALS																		
Recommendations	3–5	6–11	2–4	2–3	2–3	See note *	See note †	>58% of diet	30% of diet	<30% of diet	From food label	<10% of diet	<300 mg	3000 mg	700–900 ug	65–90 mg	See note ‡	See note §

IMPLEMENT CHANGE: NUTRITION

DAY THREE Food	Vegetable Servings	Breads and Cereals Servings	Fruit Servings	Dairy Servings	Meats and Protein Servings	Calories (kcals)	Protein (gm)	Carbohydrate (g)	Fiber (g)	Fat (g)	Total Fat % (kcal)	Saturated Fat (g)	Cholestorol (mg)	Sodium (mg)	Vitamin A (ug)	Vitamin C (mg)	Calcium (mg)	Iron (mg)
TOTALS																		
Recommendations	3–5	6–11	2–4	2–3	2–3	See note *	See note †	>58% of diet	30% of diet	<30% of diet	From food label	<10% of diet	<300 mg	3000 mg	700–900 ug	65–90 mg	See note ‡	See note §

Nutrition Plan

Once you have completed your 3-day diet assessment, look through it to identify patterns and answer the questions below.

After studying my 3-day assessment, I see that my diet is lacking in the following nutrients/food groups:

_____

_____

I can increase my intake of these nutrients/food groups by eating the following healthy, low-fat, low-sugar foods:

_____

_____

After studying my 3-day assessment, I see that my diet consists of too much of the following nutrients/food groups:

_____

_____

I can decrease my intake of these nutrients/food groups by cutting out unnecessary foods such as:

_____

_____

Fill out the behavior change contract on page 25 when you are ready to begin your new nutrition plan.

Nutrition Log

Use this log after you have developed your new nutrition plan and record what you eat each day. It will help you assess how well you are sticking to your plan.

Tip: Record information such as where you ate, what else you were doing, and your thoughts and feelings while eating in the Comments column.

DATE: _____ DAY OF WEEK: _____

Time of Day	Meal or Snack?	Food	Food Group	Serving Size	Comments

DATE: _____   DAY OF WEEK: _____

Time of Day	Meal or Snack?	Food	Food Group	Serving Size	Comments

DATE: _____   DAY OF WEEK: _____

Time of Day	Meal or Snack?	Food	Food Group	Serving Size	Comments

DATE: _____   DAY OF WEEK: _____

Time of Day	Meal or Snack?	Food	Food Group	Serving Size	Comments

MANAGING YOUR WEIGHT

Maintaining a healthy body weight is important in reducing your risk for disease and injury. Several key points for a healthy weight management program are listed below. Keep these in mind as you develop your weight management plan.

1. Determine your present weight. Calculate your body mass index (BMI) and determine if you really need to lose or gain weight.

2. Make your goals realistic. Don't try to accomplish too much too fast. Set short-term goals that you can accomplish followed by long-term goals that focus on your overall plan.

3. Eat healthfully. Move away from higher-calorie or processed foods and substitute lower-calorie, unprocessed foods.

4. Start an exercise program. Exercise burns calories, builds muscles, helps regulate blood sugar levels and appetite, reduces nervous tension, helps you cope with stress, and improves mood and self-image.

5. Recruit your friends to help. A partner makes your program easier to follow.

6. Work on your psychological well-being. Relaxing and having fun may help you resist some of the emotional drive to overeat.

7. Don't be upset by plateaus or setbacks. There will be times when you don't seem to be making progress. Or, there may be problems that prevent you from following your plan. Don't get discouraged! Problems will happen, and you must be persistent and continue your program.

8. Make long-term goals. These may be hard to pursue because you get little feedback in the short-term. Use short-term goals to help you realize the long-term goals.

9. Remember, health is the ultimate goal. Weight loss may be your focus, but if your health suffers, your long-term goal has not been achieved.

10. Log your progress. Maintaining this log book will be an essential part of your plan to record and achieve your goals.

Calculating Your BMI and BMR, and Estimating Daily Energy Expenditure

The following three parts will take you through a series of calculations that will provide an estimation of how your body expends energy. Only a specialist can give you a completely accurate reading, but these calculations can give you a general idea of what you'll need to begin a weight loss program.

Part A: Calculating Your Body Mass Index (BMI)

BMI is a useful measure of overweight and obesity that is calculated from your height and weight. It is a good gauge of your risk for diseases that can occur with more body fat, so the higher your BMI, the higher your risk is for certain diseases. If you have a high BMI, you could be at risk for heart disease, high blood pressure, type 2 diabetes, gallstones, breathing problems, and certain cancers.

BMI can be calculated using the metric or standard system. If you are using the metric system, you must express your weight in kilograms (1 kilogram = 2.2 pounds) and your height in meters (1 inch = 0.0254 meters).

BMI = body weight (kg)/(height in meters)^2

OR

BMI = [body weight (lbs)/(height in inches)^2] × 703

Your BMI = _____

- Underweight = BMI below 18.5

- Normal = BMI 18.5–24.9

- Overweight = BMI 25.0–29.9

- Obese = BMI 30.0 and above

Although BMI can be used for most men and women, it does have some limits. It may overestimate body fat in athletes and others who have a muscular build. It may also underestimate body fat in older persons and others who have lost muscle. If you need a more accurate calculation of total body fat, talk to your health care provider.

Source: The National Heart, Lung, and Blood Institute. www.nhlbi.nih.gov.

Part B: Calculating BMR and Energy Expenditure

Your basal metabolic rate (BMR) is the rate at which you burn calories to sustain life functions at rest at a normal room temperature. Your activities, fitness level, stress level, and many other things will affect your BMR.

1. Calculate your BMR (the method shown here uses the Harris-Benedict formula):

   Men:

   1. BMR = 66 + (6.3 × weight in pounds) + (12.9 × height in inches) – (6.8 × age in years)
   2. BMR = 66 + (_____) + (_____) – (_____)
   3. BMR = _____ Calories (Cal)

   Women:

   1. BMR = 655 + (4.3 × weight in pounds) + (4.7 × height in inches) – (4.7 × age in years)
   2. BMR = 655 + (_____) + (_____) – (_____)
   3. BMR = _____ Calories (Cal)

2. Estimate your total energy expenditure (EE):

Total energy expenditure takes into account your amount of activity within a 24-hour period. You can calculate your energy expenditure by keeping an activity log and adding up the calories expended during any non-sleep time. To do this, use the physical activity tracking tool on the MyPlate website (www.choosemyplate.gov). Another way to estimate total energy expenditure is to use the following calculations. Choose your level of activity on *average* and use that formula to calculate your energy expenditure (EE).

IMPLEMENT CHANGE: WEIGHT MANAGEMENT

Multiply your BMR by the appropriate activity factor, completing ONE equation below:

- If you are **sedentary** (little or no exercise)

  EE = _____ (BMR) × **1.2** = _____ Calories (Cal)

- If you are **lightly active** (light exercise/sports 1-3 days/week)

  EE = _____ (BMR) × **1.375** = _____ Calories (Cal)

- If you are **moderately active** (moderate exercise/sports 3-5 days/week)

  EE = _____ (BMR) × **1.55** = _____ Calories (Cal)

- If you are **very active** (hard exercise/sports 6-7 days/week)

  EE = _____ (BMR) × **1.725** = _____ Calories (Cal)

- If you are **extra active** (very hard daily exercise/sports & physical job or 2xday training)

  EE = _____ (BMR) × **1.9** = _____ Calories (Cal)

Source: *Get Fit, Stay Well!*, 2nd ed., by Janet Hopson, Rebecca Donatelle, and Tanya Littrell. Copyright © 2013 by Pearson Education.

Part C: Balancing Caloric Intake and Expenditure

Recall that 1 pound of fat contains approximately 3500 calories. Therefore, a negative caloric balance of 500 calories/day will result in a weight loss of 1 pound per week. Use the following formula to compute your daily caloric intake and energy expenditure that would result in a daily caloric deficit of 500 calories.

estimated daily caloric expenditure (EE) – 500 calories (deficit) = daily caloric intake needed to produce a 500-calorie deficit

In the space provided, compute your daily caloric intake needed to produce a weight loss of 1 pound per week.

_____ (estimated caloric expenditure, EE)

–500 (caloric deficit (250 caloric intake + 250 energy expenditure)) =

_____ (target daily caloric intake)

Remember: It is *always* a good idea to include exercise in your weight loss plan. The above formula suggests that your 500-calorie deficit is split evenly between eating 250 fewer calories and expending 250 more calories.

Weight Management and Exercise

- For those who want to gain weight, it is important to remember that eating more calories will cause an increase in body fat. Of course, this is undesirable. The only healthy way to gain body weight is to add muscle mass. This can be accomplished through any type of resistance training.

- Exercise must play a role in any weight management program. Exercise increases caloric expenditure both during and long after completing a workout. The table below provides information on the calories burned for selected sporting activities for a 30-minute bout of activity

Calories Burned for Selected Sporting Activities

Activity	Calories burned per 30 min
Jumping Rope	420 kcal
Jogging (7 mph)	400 kcal
Soccer	300 kcal
Singles tennis	280 kcal
Walking (4.5 mph)	230 kcal
Slow swimming	200 kcal
Leisure cycling	140 kcal
Calisthenics	130 kcal
Walking (3 mph)	120 kcal

Source: Adapted from *Health: The Basics*, 10th ed., by Rebecca Donatelle.
Copyright © 2013 by Pearson Education.

Setting Goals

It is important to set goals for your new weight management program. Refer to Section 2: Plan Change for guidelines on setting useful short-term and long-term goals. The information below may help you in forming goals for your weight management program.

My current weight is _____

I would like to weigh _____

My current total energy expenditure (EE) is _____

My current daily caloric intake is _____

My target caloric intake is _____

In order to attain my target caloric intake, I will create a caloric difference of _____ by modifying my diet and a caloric difference of _____ through exercise.

Weight Management Log

DIRECTIONS: Use the following log to track your progress.

ENTER								CALCULATE		
		Weight* (lbs)		Food (kcal)		Exercise (kcal)		Weight Diff. (lbs)	Food Diff. (kcal)	Exercise Diff. (kcal)
Date	Day	Goal	Today	Goal	Today	Goal	Today			

*Measure body weight weekly.

ENTER								CALCULATE		
		Weight* (lbs)		Food (kcal)		Exercise (kcal)		Weight Diff. (lbs)	Food Diff. (kcal)	Exercise Diff. (kcal)
Date	Day	Goal	Today	Goal	Today	Goal	Today			

*Measure body weight weekly.

IMPLEMENT CHANGE: WEIGHT MANAGEMENT

ENTER								CALCULATE		
		Weight* (lbs)		Food (kcal)		Exercise (kcal)		Weight Diff.	Food Diff.	Exercise Diff.
Date	Day	Goal	Today	Goal	Today	Goal	Today	(lbs)	(kcal)	(kcal)

*Measure body weight weekly.

PHYSICAL FITNESS

In this section of the Behavior Change Log Book, you can evaluate your fitness levels, establish fitness goals, and create an overall fitness plan. The following logs will help you track and analyze your cardiorespiratory fitness, weight training, and flexibility programs.

Benefits of Physical Fitness

When evaluating your current fitness levels and prescribing a new exercise regimen, take into account the benefits specific to cardiorespiratory fitness, muscular strength and endurance, and flexibility. Cardiorespiratory fitness decreases the risk of heart disease and diabetes, lowers blood pressure, increases bone density, and contributes to a longer life. Increased muscular strength and endurance lower the incidence of low back pain, reduce the risk of injuries, reduce the risk of osteoporosis, and improve personal appearance and self-esteem. Improved flexibility results in increased joint mobility, resistance to muscle injury, prevention of low back problems, efficient body movement, and improved posture and personal appearance. By improving all three areas of fitness, you will reap the benefits of increased health and wellness and reduce your risk for many diseases and injuries.

Components of Fitness

There are five health-related components of physical fitness. While your fitness program can focus on one of these components, ideally you should plan to include all components to maintain a healthy balance. They are:

- Cardiorespiratory endurance: the ability of your cardiovascular and respiratory systems to provide oxygen to your muscles during sustained exercise.

- Muscular strength: the ability of your muscles to exert force (i.e., lifting weight).

- Muscular endurance: the ability of your muscles to contract repeatedly over time.

- Flexibility: the ability to move your joints in a full range of motion.

- Body composition: the relative amounts of fat and lean tissue in your body.

Basic Fitness Principles

In order to design an effective fitness program, you should take into account the basic principles of fitness. These principles explain how the body responds or adapts to exercise training and, if followed correctly, will help prevent injury. While there are many fitness principles that can guide your fitness program, the following four are important. (You can read about the others in the fitness chapter of your textbook.)

- Overload: this principle states that in order to see improvements, you must make the amount of training more than the specific body system is used to.

- Progression: this principle states that in order to increase your fitness level without injury, you should increase your workout slowly. Follow the "10 percent rule," which says to increase your program frequency, intensity, or duration by no more than 10 percent per week.

- Reversibility: this principle states that if you do not maintain a minimal level of physical activity and exercise, your fitness levels will slip. Use it or lose it!

- Rest and Recovery: this principle states that in order to get the most out of your fitness program, you must schedule periods of rest and recovery. This will prevent injury and allow you to experience the full benefit of your fitness program. It is recommended that you schedule 1 to 3 rest days for cardiorespiratory training and every other day for strength training.

Physical Activity Guidelines

Creating an effective fitness program should also take into account the amount of physical activity it is recommended you do per week as well as your target heart rate.

General Physical Activity Guidelines

The General Physical Activity Guidelines are created by the U.S. Department of Health and Human Services and list the recommended amount of physical activity that adults, older adults, and children and adolescents should maintain for good health. These guidelines also include further details for these groups for additional fitness or weight loss benefits.

- Adults: To remain healthy, they should engage in 150 min/week of moderate-intensity exercise *or* 75 min/week of vigorous-intensity exercise *or* an equivalent combination of moderate- and vigorous-intensity exercise *plus* muscle strengthening activities for all major muscle groups at least 2 days/week. For additional fitness or weight loss benefits, they should engage in 300 min/week of moderate-intensity exercise *or* 150 min/week of vigorous-intensity exercise *or* an equivalent combination of moderate- and vigorous-intensity exercise *plus* muscle strengthening activities for all major muscle groups at least 2 days/week.

- Older Adults: To remain healthy, they should try to follow the same guidelines as given to adults, but if unable to, they should do as much physical activity as their physician allows. For additional fitness or weight loss benefits, they should try to follow the same guidelines as given to adults, but if unable to, they should do as much physical activity as their physician allows. For both categories, older adults should attempt muscle strengthening activities and exercises to improve balance.

- Children and Adolescents: To remain healthy, they should engage in 60 min or more of moderate- or vigorous-intensity physical activity daily *plus* muscle and bone strengthening activities within these 60 minutes at least 3 days/week. For additional fitness or weight loss benefits, they should add vigorous-intensity physical activities within the 60 daily minutes at least 3 days/week.

The FITT Principle

The FITT acronym stands for *frequency, intensity, time,* and *type;* these are all factors that should be considered while planning a personal fitness program. The exercise prescriptions for cardiorespiratory fitness, muscular fitness, and flexibility will include FITT guidelines for each.

- Frequency: the number of times per week that you exercise.

- Intensity: how hard you exercise.

- Time: how long you exercise.

- Type: what kind of exercise you do.

Your Target Heart Rate

One other element you should keep in mind when designing and executing your physical fitness program is your heart rate. If you do not make your target heart rate when exercising, you will not be getting the most benefit. The table below will help you find your target heart rate for your age group.

Age	Target HR Range (bpm)	10-sec count
18–24	139–179	23–30
25–29	135–174	22–29
30–34	132–169	22–28
35–39	129–165	21–28
40–44	125–160	21–27
45–49	122–156	20–26
50–54	118–151	20–25
55–59	114–147	19–25
60–64	110–142	18–24
65+	108–140	18–23

* Based upon the *HRmax method*, where 220 – age = HRmax, and the training zone is 70 to 90% of HRmax (moderate to vigorous). Individuals with low fitness levels should start below or at the low end of these ranges.

IMPLEMENT CHANGE: PHYSICAL FITNESS

Check Your Fitness

Determine your current fitness levels using the following tests. You may compare your fitness levels now (preprogram assessment) with your fitness levels after several months of your fitness program (post-program assessment). For information on performing and evaluating these tests, see the physical fitness chapter in your textbook.

Activity	Preprogram Assessment	Post-program Assessment
Cardiorespiratory Endurance		
3-Minute Step Test	1 minute recovery HR: _____	1 minute recovery HR: _____
1-Mile Walk Test	_____ time _____ HR	_____ time _____ HR
Muscular Strength and Endurance		
Bicep Curl	_____ 1 RM (pounds)	_____ 1 RM (pounds)
Shoulder Press	_____ 1 RM (pounds)	_____ 1 RM (pounds)
Push-up Test	_____ in 60 seconds	_____ in 60 seconds
Sit-up Test	_____ in 60 seconds	_____ in 60 seconds
Curl-up Test	_____ in 75 seconds	_____ in 75 seconds
Flexibility		
Sit and Reach Test	_____ inches	_____ inches
Shoulder Flexibility Test	_____ inches	_____ inches

Source: Adapted from *Get Fit, Stay Well!* 2nd ed., by Janet Hopson, Rebecca Donatelle, and Tanya Littrell. Copyright © 2013 by Pearson Education.

Exercise Prescriptions

Develop exercise prescriptions for cardiorespiratory fitness, weight training, and flexibility by using the logs on the following pages. Build your prescriptions using starter, slow progression, and maintenance phases. The key to these prescriptions is to slowly build up your exercise over time to avoid injury.

Cardiorespiratory Fitness Prescription

The FITT guidelines suggest the following for cardiorespiratory fitness:

Frequency: 3–5 days/week.

Intensity: 60%–90% of max heart rate.

Time: 20 to 60 minutes.

Type: Any rhythmic, continuous, large muscle group activity.

Week #	Exercise	Frequency (min/day)	Intensity (% of HRmax)	Duration (days/week)	Comments
1					
2					
3					
4					
5					
6					
7					
8					
9					
10					
11					
12					
13					
14					
15					
16					
17					
18					
19					
20					
21					
22					
23					
24					

Muscular Fitness Prescription

The FITT guidelines suggest the following for muscular fitness:

Frequency: 2–3 days/week.

Intensity: 60%–80% of resistance (1RM).

Time: 8–10 exercises, 2–4 sets, 8–12 reps.

Type: Resistance training for all major muscle groups.

Week #	Exercise	Frequency (days/week)	Weight	Sets/Reps	Comments
1					
2					
3					
4					
5					
6					
7					
8					
9					
10					
11					
12					
13					
14					
15					
16					
17					
18					
19					
20					
21					
22					
23					
24					

Flexibility Prescription

The FITT guidelines suggest the following for flexibility:

Frequency: Minimally 2–3 days per week.

Intensity: To the point of mild tension.

Time: 10–60 seconds per stretch, 4+ repetitions.

Type: Stretching, dance, or yoga exercises for all major muscle groups.

Week #	Exercise	Frequency (days/week)	Sets/Hold Time	Comments
1				
2				
3				
4				
5				
6				
7				
8				
9				
10				
11				
12				
13				
14				
15				
16				
17				
18				
19				
20				
21				
22				
23				
24				

Exercise Logs

Now, using your exercise prescriptions as guides, log your progress in your new cardiorespiratory, weight training, and flexibility programs.

Cardiorespiratory Fitness Log

DIRECTIONS: In the spaces below, keep a record of your cardiorespiratory fitness program. Exercise heart rate can be recorded as the range of heart rates measured at various times during the training session.

Date	Activity	Exercise Duration	Exercise Heart Rate	Comments

Muscular Fitness Log

DIRECTIONS: In the spaces below, record the date, number of sets, number of reps, and the weight for each exercise in your weight training program.

Date	Exercise	Sets/Reps/ Weight	Sets/Reps/ Weight	Sets/Reps/ Weight	Sets/Reps/ Weight	Sets/Reps/ Weight	Sets/Reps/ Weight	Sets/Reps/ Weight

Flexibility Log

DIRECTIONS: In the spaces below, record the date, sets, and hold time for each exercise in your flexibility program.

Date	Exercise	Sets/Hold Time	Sets/Hold Time	Sets/Hold Time	Sets/Hold Time	Sets/Hold Time	Sets/Hold Time	Sets/Hold Time

4 Evaluate Change

WEEKLY BEHAVIOR CHANGE EVALUATION

This worksheet will allow you to keep track of where you are in your behavior change project on a weekly basis. While there are only four copies of this worksheet here, you can find more in the behavior change section of your textbook companion website.

NAME: _____ DATE: _____

DIRECTIONS: Answer the following questions for each week of your behavior change project, and be sure to save them for your final evaluation of the entire project.

1. What was your goal for this behavior change project?

_____

_____

_____

2. What was your goal for the week?

_____

_____

_____

3. Did you keep a journal of your behavior?

_____

_____

_____

4. What did your journal reveal about your behavior?

_____

_____

_____

5. What other observations did your partner or instructor see in your journal?

_____

_____

_____

6. Did you achieve your weekly goal? Did you give yourself a reward for success?

_____

_____

_____

7. What contributed to your success or failure?

_____

_____

_____

8. What goal will you set for next week?

_____

_____

_____

9. How will you reward yourself next week?

_____

_____

_____

10. What are you learning about yourself with this self-management project?

_____

_____

_____

NAME: _____ DATE: _____

DIRECTIONS: Answer the following questions for each week of your behavior change project and for the final evaluation of your entire project.

1. What was your goal for this behavior change project?

_____

_____

_____

2. What was your goal for the week?

_____

_____

_____

3. Did you keep a journal of your behavior?

_____

_____

_____

4. What did your journal reveal about your behavior?

_____

_____

_____

5. What other observations did your partner or instructor see in your journal?

_____

_____

_____

6. Did you achieve your weekly goal? Did you give yourself a reward for success?

_____

_____

_____

7. What contributed to your success or failure?

_____

_____

_____

8. What goal will you set for next week?

_____

_____

_____

9. How will you reward yourself next week?

_____

_____

_____

10. What are you learning about yourself with this self-management project?

_____

_____

_____

NAME:_____ DATE:_____

DIRECTIONS: Answer the following questions for each week of your behavior change project and for the final evaluation of your entire project.

1. What was your goal for this behavior change project?

   _____

   _____

   _____

2. What was your goal for the week?

   _____

   _____

   _____

3. Did you keep a journal of your behavior?

   _____

   _____

   _____

4. What did your journal reveal about your behavior?

   _____

   _____

   _____

5. What other observations did your partner or instructor see in your journal?

   _____

   _____

   _____

6. Did you achieve your weekly goal? Did you give yourself a reward for success?

   _____

   _____

   _____

7. What contributed to your success or failure?

_____

_____

_____

8. What goal will you set for next week?

_____

_____

_____

9. How will you reward yourself next week?

_____

_____

_____

10. What are you learning about yourself with this self-management project?

_____

_____

_____

NAME: _____ DATE: _____

DIRECTIONS: Answer the following questions for each week of your behavior change project and for the final evaluation of your entire project.

1. What was your goal for this behavior change project?

_____

_____

_____

2. What was your goal for the week?

_____

_____

_____

3. Did you keep a journal of your behavior?

_____

_____

_____

4. What did your journal reveal about your behavior?

_____

_____

_____

5. What other observations did your partner or instructor see in your journal?

_____

_____

_____

6. Did you achieve your weekly goal? Did you give yourself a reward for success?

_____

_____

_____

7. What contributed to your success or failure?

_____

_____

_____

8. What goal will you set for next week?

_____

_____

_____

9. How will you reward yourself next week?

_____

_____

_____

10. What are you learning about yourself with this self-management project?

_____

_____

_____

REFLECTIONS

Use this worksheet to reflect on your behavior change project. Be sure to refer back to your weekly evaluation worksheets and journal entries to get an accurate picture of your progress!

NAME: _____ DATE: _____

1. My behavior change was:

   _____

   _____

2. My personal feelings on the project and behavior change process were:

   _____

   _____

3. My major obstacles and resources I used to overcome or prevent them were:

   _____

   _____

   _____

4. Summary of goals I attained:

   _____

   _____

   _____

5. My overall assessment of the assignment:

   _____

   _____

   _____

PROJECT EVALUATION

Use the following checklist to track your progress and make sure that you've completed all the necessary behavior change worksheets and assignments in this log book.

NAME: _____ DATE: _____

Behavior Change Requirement	Yes	No	Comments
• How Healthy Are You?	_____	_____	_____
• Personalizing the Six Dimensions of Health	_____	_____	_____
• Common Target Behaviors	_____	_____	_____
• Your Target Behaviors	_____	_____	_____
• Understanding Your Target Behavior: Is it Addictive?	_____	_____	_____
• Understanding Your Target Behavior: What Are Its Health Effects?	_____	_____	_____
• Understanding Your Target Behavior: Monitoring Your Behavior	_____	_____	_____
• Set Goals, Timelines, and Rewards	_____	_____	_____
• Examining Attitudes and Developing Strategies Worksheet	_____	_____	_____
• Behavior Change Contract	_____	_____	_____
• Lifelong Behavior Change Contract	_____	_____	_____
• Goal Log	_____	_____	_____
• Day One Journal Entry	_____	_____	_____
• Weeks 1–2 Journal Entry	_____	_____	_____
• Middle of Project Journal Entry	_____	_____	_____
• End of Project Journal Entry	_____	_____	_____
• Weekly Behavior Change Evaluation	_____	_____	_____
• Reflection Worksheet	_____	_____	_____